What's So Special About Manuka Honey? Book of Recipes

by Ann Adair

Table of Contents

1. Manuka Honey Butter Truffles
2. Manuka Honey Orange Ginger Smoothie
3. Manuka Honey Pecan Pistachio Parfait
4. Manuka Honey Spiced Pumpkin Bread
5. Manuka Honey Sriracha Tofu
6. Banana Pancakes with Manuka Honey Butter
7. Sage, Manuka Honey and Lemon Tea
8. Manuka Honey Sesame Winter Salad
9. Oat Pecan & Manuka Honey Breakfast Bars
10. Manuka Honey Hummus & Pita Wedges
11. Manuka Honey Cinnamon Cookies
12. Manuka Honey Cashew Butter Banana Muffins
13. Egg Salad Bagels with Manuka Honey Roasted Bacon

14. **Manuka Honey-Sweetened Brioche Grilled Cheese**

15. **Baked Manuka Honey Bacon Benedict**

16. **Honey Oatmeal Apple Cinnamon Muffins**

17. **Manuka Honey Blueberry and Passion Fruit Cupcakes**

18. **Manuka Honey Ginger Pork Ribs**

19. **Smoky Honey Lemon Garlic Cornish Hens**

20. **Strawberry Manuka Honey Lemon Popsicles**

21. **Creamy Manuka Honey Avocado Cocoa Popsicles**

22. **Mango Almond Coconut Manuka Honey Popsicles**

23. **Peanut Butter and Raspberry Popsicles**

24. **Manuka Honey Popcorn**

25. **Waffles with Honey Cream and Grilled Peaches**

26. **Manuka Honey and Pear Rice Pudding**

27. **Manuka Honey Almond Chocolate Cake**

28. **Manuka Honey Catnip Bites**

29. **Manuka Honey-Mustard Chicken and Potato Casserole**

30. **Manuka Honey Ginger Parsnip Bake**

31. **Manuka Honey Glazed Pineapple Ham**

32. **Caramelized Brussel Sprouts with Apples and Pecans**

33. **Manuka Honey Fig Dip with Fresh Garlic Pitas**

34. **Manuka Honey Spiced Carrot Cake**

35. **Manuka Honey and Thyme Cornbread**

36. **Manuka Honey Raspberry Bundt Cake**

37. **Vanilla and Manuka Honey Homemade Ice Cream**

1. Manuka Honey Butter Truffles

Ingredients:

- 2/3 cup rolled oats
- ½ cup Manuka Honey
- 1/3 cup peanut butter or almond butter
- ¼ cup ground almonds
- ½ ounce ground flaxseed
- 2 tablespoons cocoa powder
- 1 teaspoon ground cinnamon

Directions:

1. In a food processor equipped with a metal blade, or a blender, combine rolled oats, Manuka honey, ground flaxseed, cocoa powder, and cinnamon. Pulse the mixture for one to two minutes until ingredients begin to combine but are not completely mixed together.
2. Add peanut or almond butter to the food processor with the other ingredients. Turn on the food processor and allow it to run and mix the ingredients until they all have been well incorporated, and the mixture has a breadcrumb like texture.
3. Take one tablespoon of the mixture, place it in hand, and roll into a ball. If the mixture is too crumbly, add more honey and mix again in the food processor.
4. Roll the mixture into one tablespoon balls until all the mixture has been used.
5. Store the truffles in an airtight container at room temperature, or in the fridge for up to a week.

2. Manuka Honey Orange Ginger Smoothie

Ingredients:

- 1 whole carrot, washed but not peeled
- 1 whole orange, peeled
- 1 tablespoon of Manuka Honey
- 1 small piece of ginger
- juice from 1/2 a lime
- 1 cup ice
- 1 cup water

Directions:

- Put all ingredients into a blender and mix until combined and smooth.
- Pour into a glass. Enjoy!

3. Manuka Honey Pecan Pistachio Parfait

Ingredients:

- 1 chopped apple or ripe pear
- 8 oz. coconut yogurt
- 5 tbsp. chopped dried fig
- 2 tbsp. chopped pecans
- 2 tbsp. chopped pistachios
- 2 tbsp. Manuka Honey

Directions:

In two small glasses, make alternating layers starting with chopped apple/pear at the bottom, then yogurt, then mixed dried figs and nuts and a drizzle of honey, then another layer of yogurt. Repeat the layers until all ingredients are used, ending with a dollop of yogurt on top. Enjoy!

4. Manuka Honey Spiced Pumpkin Bread

Ingredients:

- 1/3 cup melted coconut oil
- 1/2 cup Manuka Honey
- 2 eggs
- 1/4 cup hot water
- 1 teaspoon vanilla extract
- 1 cup pumpkin puree
- 1/2 teaspoon Sea Salt
- 1/2 teaspoon cinnamon
- 1/2 teaspoon ginger
- 1/4 teaspoon nutmeg
- 1/4 teaspoon cloves
- 1 cup whole wheat flour
- 3/4 cup all-purpose flour
- 1/4 tsp baking powder
- 1 teaspoon baking soda

Directions:

Preheat oven to 325 degrees F. Grease a 9×5 inch loaf pan. In a large bowl mix oil, Manuka Honey, eggs, water and vanilla together. Stir in pumpkin puree. In another bowl whisk together salt, cinnamon, ginger, nutmeg, cloves, flours, baking powder, and baking soda. Mix all ingredients together. Pour into loaf pan. Sprinkle with toasted coconut. Bake for 60 to 65 minutes. Insert a toothpick in the top to check if bread is done. It should come out clean. Let the bread cool in the loaf pan for 5 minutes, then transfer it to a wire rack.

5. Manuka Honey Sriracha Tofu

Ingredients:

- 14 ounces, fluid Firm Tofu
- 4 cloves Minced Garlic
- 4 Tablespoons Sriracha
- 4 Tablespoons Soy Sauce or Braggs Liquid Amino Acids
- 3 Tablespoons Manuka Honey
- 2 Tablespoons Rice Vinegar
- 2 Tablespoons Vegetable Oil
- 1 teaspoon Sesame Oil
- 1 Tablespoon Sesame Seeds
- 1 Scallion, Finely Chopped

Directions:

Drain tofu and wrap in paper towel to remove excess water. Slice tofu into about 1-inch cubes.

Mix garlic, Sriracha, soy sauce, honey and vinegar together with a fork to break up the firm Manuka honey, and get all ingredients combined nicely. Set aside.

Heat a medium skillet or sauce pan over high heat and add vegetable oil. When the oil is hot, add tofu cubes. Fry on each side for 2–3 minutes without touching or tossing too much, until golden brown.

Add Sriracha honey sauce and gently coat tofu cubes. Cook for an additional 3 minutes on medium heat.

Remove from heat and top with sesame oil and sesame seeds. Gently give it one last gentle stir to evenly coat tofu cubes and serve topped with scallions. Be gentle so the tofu does not fall apart. Enjoy!

6. Banana Pancakes with Manuka Honey Butter

Ingredients:

- ½ cup unsalted butter, softened
- 1/4 cup manuka honey, plus extra, to serve
- 4 bananas
- 1 cup ricotta
- 3/4 cup buttermilk
- 3 eggs, separated
- 1 1/2 cups self-rising flour
- 1/2 tsp baking powder
- 2 tbsp coconut sugar
- 2 tbsp rice bran oil
- 1/4 cup roughly chopped toasted walnuts, to serve

Directions:

1. To make the manuka honey butter, place the butter and honey in a bowl and, using a fork, mix until well combined. Place on a piece of plastic wrap and form into a log, twisting ends of wrap to secure tightly, then chill until firm.
2. Mash 2 bananas in a large bowl. Add the ricotta, buttermilk and egg yolks, and stir to combine. Sift the flour and baking powder into a separate bowl, then add the sugar. Add the flour mixture to the banana mixture and stir to combine. Whisk the egg whites to stiff peaks. Gently fold one-third of the egg white into the batter to loosen, then fold in the remainder.
3. Heat 1 tbsp oil in a frying pan over medium heat. Working in batches, add 1/4-cup portions of batter to the pan and cook for 2-3 minutes each side until golden, adding more oil to the pan between batches, if necessary. Remove from the pan and keep warm while cooking the remainder.
4. Slice the remaining 2 bananas on an angle. Stack the pancakes on a platter and top with slices of honey butter, banana and chopped

walnut, if using. Serve with extra honey. Enjoy!

7. Sage, Manuka Honey and Lemon Tea

Ingredients:

- 12 fresh sage leaves
- Boiling water
- Juice of ½ lemon
- 2 teaspoons Raw Manuka Honey

Directions:

1. In a cup pop in 12 fresh sage leaves, add boiling water, cover and leave to infuse for approximately 20 minutes.
2. Remove the sage leaves and add juice of 1/2 lemon and 2 teaspoons Raw Manuka Honey. Drink while still warm. Enjoy!

8. Manuka Honey Sesame Winter Salad

Ingredients:

- ¼ red cabbage
- ¼ white cabbage
- 4 leaves of kale
- 2 large carrots
- 2 spring onions
- 2 garlic cloves, sliced
- 1 tbsp. white wine vinegar
- 3-4 tbsp. Organic Olive Oil
- 1 tsp. grain mustard
- 1 tbsp. Manuka Honey
- 1 handful mixed seeds –sesame and sunflower
- Small handful fresh mint

Directions:

1. Finely shred the cabbages.
2. Roughly chop the kale excluding stocks.
3. Peel and finely slice the carrots.
4. Finely slice the spring onions.
5. Place in a large bowl.
6. Gently fry the garlic in a little olive oil. Do not burn.
7. In a food processor, add the fried garlic, vinegar, oil and mustard and blend for a few minutes, then stop and add the Manuka Honey.

8. Blend for a few seconds.

9. Add a pinch of sea salt and black pepper, then pour it over the sliced vegetables.

10. Use your clean hands to toss and dress everything.

11. Heat the seeds in a dry pan for a few minutes until warm, then scatter them over the salad.

12. Pick and tear over your mint leaves. Consume immediately.

9. Oat Pecan & Manuka Honey Breakfast Bars

Ingredients:

1 cup porridge oats

1 cup pecan halves

10 dates chopped finely

½ cup pumpkin seeds

2 teaspoons cinnamon

1 teaspoon sea salt

1 tablespoon maple syrup

2 tablespoons manuka honey

1 tablespoon light olive oil

2 tablespoons melted butter

Directions:

Preheat oven to 350°F. Blend ingredients together in a bowl with a fork and mash until well mixed. Spread in the bottom of a non-stick or foil lined small baking tray (6 x 8 inches or smaller). Bars should be about 1 inch thick. Bake for about 30 minutes. Let cool and slice. Enjoy!

10. Manuka Honey Hummus & Pita Wedges

Ingredients:

Hummus:

- 1 cup drained, rinsed, cooked chickpeas
- 5 cloves garlic, roasted
- 1/2 cup olive oil
- 1/2 cup tahini
- 2 tablespoons Manuka Honey
- 1/2 teaspoon ground cumin
- 1/2 teaspoon salt
- Juice of 2 lemons

Garlic pita wedges:

- 4 small pitta pockets
- 1/2 cup parsley, finely chopped
- 2 cloves garlic, crushed
- 1/4 cup olive oil
- 1 ½ Tblsp. butter, softly melted

Directions:

1. For the Hummus: Place all the Hummus ingredients into a food processor and blend until smooth.
2. Garnish with sweet paprika and a drizzle of olive oil.
3. For the Wedges: Preheat oven to 425 degrees F.
4. Cut pita pocket in half, length ways.
5. Mix all ingredients together in a cup and Spread mixture evenly all over pita.

6. Toast the pita pockets in the oven approximately 3 minutes or until golden and crispy. Enjoy!

11. Manuka Honey Cinnamon Cookies

Yield: 12 cookies

Ingredients:

- 1 stick plus 2.5 tablespoons of salted butter, softened
- ⅔ cup of sugar
- 4 tablespoons of Manuka honey
- 1 teaspoon of cinnamon
- 1 egg
- Lime zest
- ½ teaspoon of baking powder
- 1 ⅔ cups of flour

Directions:

1. To begin, set your oven to preheat to 350 degrees Fahrenheit.
2. After providing enough time for the butter to soften, beat your butter and your sugar in a medium-sized bowl until a lighter and creamy paste has formed.
3. Now, add the Manuka honey, the cinnamon, the egg, and the lime zest into the mix, blending well.
4. In a separate bowl, mix the flour and the baking powder together, and then toss the powdered mixture into your batter, mixing it well.
5. Find a suitable and clean flat surface, and then spread some extra flour over it, so you can extend the dough. Using a cookie cutter of your choice, cut out your cookies.
6. Once all your dough has been used, place the cookies on an uncovered, un-greased baking sheet and take them to your oven, baking for about 10 minutes or until they have browned slightly. Allow the cookies some time to cool on a cooling rack or on some wax paper before serving. Enjoy!

12. Manuka Honey Cashew Butter Banana Muffins

Ingredients:

- ½ cup of sultanas
- 1 and 1/4 heaping cups of flour, self-raising
- ¼ cup of oats
- 1 teaspoon of baking powder
- 2 eggs
- ½ cup of Manuka Honey
- 2 bananas, mashed
- ½ cup of cashew butter
- ¼ cup of butter, melted
- ¾ cup plus 1/8 cup of milk

Directions:

1. To begin, preheat your oven to 375 degrees Fahrenheit, and then place 12 paper muffin baking cups into a muffin tray or spray the muffin tray's cups with cooking spray.
2. In a large enough bowl, mix the sultanas, the flour, the oats, and the baking powder before setting to the side.
3. In a separate bowl, beat in the eggs before gently beating in the Manuka honey, bananas, melted butter, milk, and cashew butter.
4. In your dry ingredients bowl, make a well at the center before pouring the wet ingredients in, combining quickly. Avoid over mixing – the wet and dry ingredients only have to be combined, so stop mixing once no dry flour is visible.
5. Spoon the batter into the cups of your muffin tray and bake between 25 and 30 minutes until the tops of the muffins are a golden-brown color. Allow the muffins to cool down on a cooling rack. Enjoy!

13. Egg Salad Bagels with Manuka Honey Roasted Bacon

Ingredients:

- 2 bagels, sliced
- 1 or 2 tablespoons of Manuka Honey
- 6 slices of bacon, thick cut
- 4 eggs
- 1/2 teaspoon of mustard
- 3 tablespoons of mayonnaise
- 2 tablespoons of bell pepper, diced finely
- 1 tablespoon of red onion, grated or minced finely
- 2 tablespoons of carrots, shredded
- 1 tablespoon of parsley or cilantro, chopped
- Pepper and salt to taste
- 2 slices of cheese

Directions:

1. Start by preheating your oven to 400 degrees Fahrenheit.
2. Place your thick cut bacon onto a rack that is set over an aluminum-foil lined baking sheet. Drizzle the bacon with the Manuka honey before placing it into your oven for 15 or 20 minutes.
3. Bring a larger pot of water up to a boil before adding your eggs. Cook them on high heat for about 10 minutes before taking them off the heat and running them under cold water. Then, peel your eggs and chop them into smaller pieces.
4. In a medium-sized bowl, combine the mustard and mayonnaise before adding the chopped eggs, along with the bell pepper, the red onion, the shredded carrots, and the parsley or cilantro. Stir the ingredients until they are just combined, seasoning with pepper and salt to taste.

5. For properly assembling this sandwich, take your bagels and lightly toast them, placing one slice of cheese onto each bottom half. Once your bagels are ready, top the cheese with the Manuka honey bacon and egg salad. Enjoy!

14. Manuka Honey-Sweetened Brioche Grilled Cheese

Ingredients for Brioche Grilled Cheese:

Manuka Honey Bacon Jam:

- 1 teaspoon of butter
- 2 pieces of diced bacon
- 1/2 an onion, diced
- 1/4 teaspoon of black pepper
- 2 tablespoons of Manuka honey

Rosemary-Infused Manuka Honey:

- 1 sprig of rosemary
- 1/4 cup of Manuka honey

Brioche Grilled Cheese:

- 4 slices of brioche bread
- 1 tablespoon of butter
- 2 tablespoons of Manuka honey bacon jam
- 1/4 cup of rosemary-infused Manuka honey
- 1/4 lb. of sliced Taleggio cheese

Directions for Brioche Grilled Cheese:

1. **Manuka Honey Bacon Jam:** Using a large sauté pan, melt the butter and spread it around your pan, and then add the bacon and onions

over low-medium heat. For about 15 minutes, cook your bacon and onions, stirring every now and then until they have caramelized.

2. Add the black pepper and Manuka honey, cooking for another 3 minutes. Remove the pan from the heat, allowing the contents to cool before continuing. Puree in a food processor until smooth, reserving later for your sandwiches.

3. **Rosemary-Infused Manuka Honey**: Using a smaller sauce pan, heat the rosemary and the Manuka honey for about 2 minutes before removing from the heat. Allow the flavors to fully infuse, about 10 minutes, before transferring to a smaller bowl and reserving for your sandwiches.

4. **Brioche Grilled Cheese:** On one side for each slice of brioche bread, spread an even layer of butter. Layer on the Taleggio cheese as well as 1 tablespoon of Manuka honey bacon jam onto 2 pieces before topping with the second piece.

5. Heat a skillet or pan, and then, over lower heat, sear the sandwiches until the brioche has browned and the cheese has melted. Flip and repeat on the other side. Slice the sandwiches in half on diagonals (for dipping purpose) before serving with the rosemary-infused Manuka honey. Enjoy!

15. Baked Manuka Honey Bacon Benedict

Ingredients:

- 1 package of 6-8 split English muffins
- 4 tablespoons of butter
- 1 lb. of thicker bacon
- 12 eggs
- 1/4 cup of Manuka honey
- Salt and pepper for flavor

For the Hollandaise:

- 1 one stick of butter
- 2 cups of 2 percent milk
- 2 packages of hollandaise sauce
- Fresh paprika and chives or parsley for the garnish

Directions:

1. Preheat your oven on Bake to 350 degrees Fahrenheit.
2. On each muffin half, spread butter and then bake for about 10 minutes on a baking sheet. Set to the side.
3. Next, spread out the bacon on a pan lined with parchment, drizzling the Manuka honey on the bacon. Bake the bacon for about 20 or 25 minutes, turning over once. Move each bacon slice to a cooling rack for cooling and draining. Cut every bacon piece in half.
4. Now, prepare your hollandaise sauce as per your packaging directions, keeping it warm while preparing the rest of the meal.
5. Place each muffin half on a baking sheet, evenly dividing the bacon slices over every muffin half. Lightly break open a single egg over each individual muffin half, sprinkling with pepper and salt for

flavor. From here, bake the bacon benedict between 12-15 minutes or when the eggs are cooked to your personal preference.

Serve immediately, topped with your warm hollandaise while garnishing with herbs and a pinch of paprika. Enjoy!

16. Honey Oatmeal Apple Cinnamon Muffins

Ingredients:

- 2/3 cup of whole wheat flour
- 1 cup of all-purpose flour
- 1 teaspoon of baking soda
- 1 teaspoon of baking powder
- 1/2 teaspoon of salt
- 1 teaspoon of cinnamon, heaping
- 1 egg
- 1/2 cup of Manuka honey
- 1/3 cup of vegetable oil
- 1 1/2 teaspoon of vanilla extract
- 1/2 cup of milk
- 1/3 cup of old fashioned oats
- 1 1/2 cups of apples, thinly diced

Directions:

1. Preheat your oven on bake to 350 degrees Fahrenheit. Then, place 12 liners into a cupcake/muffin pan.
2. In a big enough bowl, whisk the flours, baking soda, baking powder, salt, and cinnamon together.
3. In another mixing bowl, whisk the egg, Manuka honey, oil, vanilla extract, and milk. Add the bowl's contents to the dry ingredient mixture, stirring gently until the contents are just combined. Try not to over mix everything.
4. Pour the oats and the apples into the bowl, gently folding them into the mixture.
5. Now, divide up the muffin batter consistently amongst the 12 muffin cups.

6. Finally, bake the muffins for 18-20 minutes in your preheated oven or until a centered, inserted toothpick comes up clean. Let them cool before serving. Enjoy!

17. Manuka Honey Blueberry and Passion Fruit Cupcakes

Ingredients:

- 2 cups of all-purpose flour, unbleached
- 1/2 teaspoon of baking powder
- 1/2 teaspoon of baking soda
- 1/2 teaspoon of salt
- 1/4 cup of buttermilk
- 3/4 cup of passion fruit nectar
- 1/2 cup of softened butter
- 2 large eggs
- 1/2 cup of Manuka honey
- 1 cup (or 8 oz.) of fresh blueberries

For Passion Fruit Manuka Honey Whipped Cream:

- 2 tablespoons of passion fruit nectar
- 1 cup of heavy whipping cream
- 1 tablespoon of Manuka honey

Directions:

1. Set out one stick of butter a few hours before you start baking.
2. For the passion fruit Manuka honey whipped cream, combine the whipping cream, passion fruit nectar, and Manuka honey in a small mixing bowl. Beat the mixture until peaks eventually form.
3. For the cupcakes, preheat the oven to 350 degrees Fahrenheit. Sift the flour, baking powder, baking soda, and salt together. Then, set aside.
4. In a measuring cup for liquids, combine the buttermilk and passion fruit nectar, and then set to the aside.

5. In a larger mixing bowl, cream the butter until it is fluffy. Add the Manuka honey afterward and mix it well. Add the eggs, one at a time, whisking each. Now, add half of your earmarked dry mixture over into the butter mixture – mix until it is just combined.
6. With your mixer running on a low setting, gradually add in the passion fruit mix. (You can hand mix this if you prefer.)
7. Now, add in the rest of the dry ingredients until they are just combined. Lightly fold the blueberries in. In a muffin/cupcake tray, fill 12-14 paper-lined muffin cups 2/3 of the way full. Bake for 18-22 minutes or when a toothpick pushed into a muffin's center comes out spotless. Set the cupcakes on a wire rack to cool. Then, frost them with the passion fruit Manuka honey whipped cream. Enjoy!

18. Manuka Honey Ginger Pork Ribs

Ingredients:

- 2 (2 to 2.5 lb.) slabs of pork ribs
- 2 teaspoons fresh ground pepper
- 1 tablespoon kosher salt
- 1/2 cups Manuka honey
- 2 tablespoons Asian chili-garlic sauce
- 2 tablespoons soy sauce
- 1 tablespoon butter
- 1 tablespoon lime juice
- 1 teaspoon ground ginger
- 1 teaspoon dry mustard

Directions:

1. Preheat the oven to 325 degrees Fahrenheit.
2. Rinse the slabs and then pat them dry. Remove the skinny membrane from the back of the slabs by cutting into it before then pulling it out. This will make the pork ribs a bit more tender.
3. Sprinkle pepper and salt over the slabs and then wrap each of the slabs in tight aluminum foil. Set the slabs onto a jelly-roll pan, baking them for 2 to 2 ½ hours, or when they are tender, and the meat pulls from the bone.
4. Mix the Manuka honey, Asian chill-garlic sauce, soy sauce, butter, lime juice, ginger, and dry mustard in a saucepan and bring it to boil on high heat, occasionally stirring. Reduce the heat down to medium-low and simmer for 5 minutes or when it's reduced by half. Move the mixture over into a bowl.
5. Remove the ribs from the oven. Raise the temperature of the oven to broil on high. Remove the slabs from the foil carefully and then place them on a baking sheet lined with aluminum foil. Brush both rib slabs with 3 tablespoons of the Manuka honey mixture each.

6. Broil for 5-7 minutes or when the slabs are sticky and browned. Brush them with the last of the Manuka honey mixture. Enjoy!

19. Smoky Honey Lemon Garlic Cornish Hens

Ingredients:

- 4 fresh Cornish hens
- 1 lemon, quartered
- Juice from 2 large lemons
- 1 tablespoon each — basil, thyme, rosemary, and oregano, dried and crushed
- 4 tablespoons Manuka honey
- 1 tablespoon coarse black pepper
- 3 tablespoons butter
- 1/4 cup low sodium soy sauce
- 1 teaspoon liquid smoke
- 4 large cloves of garlic
- 1-1/2 dozen small red potatoes, washed

Directions:

1. Preheat the oven for 350 degrees F. Clean and rinse the inside cavity of the four Cornish hens.
2. Place the hens in a large oven proof baking dish. Then, tie the legs together and tuck the wings under.
3. Insert a 1/4 lemon and a large clove of garlic in the cavity of each hen.
4. Set the potatoes in a bowl, seasoning with 2 tablespoons of olive oil and half of the herbs. Place the seasoned potatoes in the pan around the hens.
5. Cover the pan with loose aluminum foil and then bake for about 30 minutes. Add the rest of the herbs, the black pepper, lemon juice, butter, Manuka honey, soy sauce, and liquid smoke to a small sauce pan. Simmer the pan over a low flame, stir continuously for 5 minutes, and then remove the pan from the heat.

6. Remove the hens from the oven and then baste them with the soy sauce mixture. Return the hens to the oven and bake them for an extra 10 minutes.
7. Remove the hens from the oven, repeating the basting/baking process for another 20 minutes or when the hens are ready.
8. Test the hens to see if they are done by pushing a fork into the thickest part of each hen. If the liquid runs clear, then your hens are ready. Enjoy!

20. Strawberry Manuka Honey Lemon Popsicles

Ingredients:

- 3 cups fresh (or frozen, thawed) strawberries, hulled and halved
- 3 tablespoons fresh lemon juice
- 1/2 cup Manuka honey

Directions:

1. Using a food processor, blend the strawberries, lemon juice, and Manuka honey until smooth.
2. Pour the puree into molds or cups with wooden spoons at the middle of each.
3. Freeze the Popsicles until they are solid.

21. Creamy Manuka Honey Avocado Cocoa Popsicles

Ingredients:

- 1 large, ripe avocado, peel and pit discarded
- ½ cup Manuka honey
- 1/3 cup cocoa powder
- 1 1/3 cup unsweetened vanilla almond milk
- Pinch of salt

Directions:

1. Place all the ingredients into a blender and blend until the mixture is completely smooth.
2. Pour the mixture into a couple of pop molds and freeze overnight or until they have completely frozen.
3. Remove them from their molds by carefully running hot water on the outside of the mold for 20-30 seconds.

22. Mango Almond Coconut Manuka Honey Popsicles

Ingredients:

- 6 cups slightly thawed frozen mango
- 1/4 cup light coconut milk
- 2 tablespoons orange juice
- 2 tablespoons Manuka honey
- 1 teaspoon vanilla extract

Directions:

1. Blend the mango, orange juice, coconut milk, Manuka honey, and vanilla extract until smooth. Fill the ice-pop molds and then freeze.

23. Peanut Butter and Raspberry Popsicles

Ingredients:

- 1/2 cup unsalted smooth peanut butter
- 1 cup low-fat plain yogurt
- 1 cup skim milk
- 3 tablespoons Manuka honey
- 2 teaspoons pure vanilla extract
- 1 1/2 cups fresh raspberries
- 2 cups unsweetened raspberry juice
- 4 tablespoons sesame seeds

Directions:

1. Using a blender, add peanut butter, milk, yogurt, vanilla extract, and 2 tablespoons of Manuka honey. Blend the ingredients until smooth.
2. Fill the Popsicle molds partially with the peanut butter mixture and freeze it for an hour.
3. Again, fill the Popsicle molds part way with raspberry juice and some raspberries. Insert the sticks and freeze the molds for an hour.
4. One more time, fill the molds with the remaining peanut butter mixture. Freeze overnight or for at least 8 hours.
5. Take the Popsicles out of the freezer and let them stand for a few minutes at room temperature before taking them out of the molds.
6. Add in the remaining Manuka honey at the bottom of each treat and coat them with sesame seeds. Enjoy!

24. Manuka Honey Popcorn

Ingredients:

- 3/4 tsp. canola oil
- 2 tbsp. mushroom popcorn kernels
- 7 tsp. sugar
- 4 tsp. Manuka honey
- 1 tsp. glucose syrup
- 1 tbsp. water
- 1 tbsp. butter
- 1⁄4 tsp. kosher salt

Directions:

1. To begin, spray a mixing bowl as well as a baking sheet lined with parchment paper with non-stick cooking spray.
2. Heat canola oil in a saucepan over medium heat. Add the popcorn kernels, cover the saucepan, and continue cooking, shaking the pan frequently until the kernels are mostly popped.
3. Transfer the popped corn to the sprayed-down mixing bowl.
4. In another saucepan, cook the sugar, water, Manuka honey, butter, and glucose syrup over medium heat, without stirring the mixture, until it becomes a deep color of amber. Then, add the salt to the mixture.
5. At this point, pour the Manuka honey caramel over the popcorn and stir to coat.
6. Pour the Manuka honey corn out onto the prepared baking tray.
7. Quickly and gently separate the popcorn while it is still warm. Enjoy!

25. Waffles with Honey Cream and Grilled Peaches

Ingredients:

Waffles:

- 1 cup and 2 teaspoons plain flour
- ½ teaspoon salt
- 3 teaspoons baking powder
- ½ teaspoon ground cinnamon
- 2 eggs, separated
- 1 and 3/4 cups milk
- 1 orange, finely grated zest
- 6 tablespoons and 2 teaspoons butter, melted, and extra for greasing

Peaches:

- 6 ripe golden-fleshed peaches
- 3 tablespoons butter, melted
- ½ teaspoon vanilla extract
- 2 tablespoons Manuka honey, extra to drizzle

Cream:

- 1 and 1/4 cup cream
- 1 teaspoon vanilla extract
- 1 tablespoon Manuka honey

Directions:

1. **To make the waffles,** sift the flour, baking powder, salt, cinnamon, and sugar in a well-sized bowl.
2. Lightly beat the egg yolks with the milk and add the mixture to the dry ingredients and with the orange zest, mixing it all into a smooth batter. Then, stir in the butter.
3. Beat the egg whites into stiff peaks, and then fold them into the batter.
4. **For the peaches,** cut them in quarters or, depending on the size, into eighths, discarding the stones. Combine the butter, the Manuka honey, and the vanilla. Add in the sliced peaches and then toss it to coat.
5. Oil down a preheated grill pan or barbecue and set the peaches with the cut side down. Cook for 3-4 minutes until the peaches are caramelized. Turn them and repeat the process on the opposite side.
6. **To make the honey cream,** take the cream and beat it until it starts to thicken. Then, add the Manuka honey and vanilla and beat until the cream thickens.
7. When the dish is ready and fit to serve, cook the batter in a waffling iron or pan, making around 12 waffles and preserving their warmth inside the oven while working.
8. Serve the waffles with a solid dollop of honey cream, a serving of peach slices, and a good drizzle of Manuka honey. Enjoy!

26. Manuka Honey and Pear Rice Pudding

Ingredients:

- ¼ cup and 3 tablespoons of pudding rice
- 2 ½ cups of dairy milk (or almond milk for a lighter dish)
- 4 gently crushed cardamom
- 3 tablespoons Manuka honey

For the roasted pears:

- 4 sprigs of thyme
- 2 bay leaves
- 2-4 pears, halved
- Several turns of black freshly ground pepper
- A drizzle of olive oil
- A generous drizzle of Manuka honey

Directions:

1. Add the pudding rice to a saucepan with the cardamom, milk, and Manuka honey. Stir the ingredients occasionally.
2. Allow to cook over medium to low heat for 45 minutes to an hour.
3. Prepare the pears and drizzle them with oil, Manuka honey, seasoning, and the fresh herbs.
4. Roast for about 30-40 minutes until soft and slightly dark around the edges.
5. Once the pears and everything else is cooked, serve together. Enjoy!

27. Manuka Honey Almond Chocolate Cake

Ingredients:

- 11 tablespoons unsalted butter
- 1 ½ cup dark chocolate
- 1/3 cup + 4 teaspoons Manuka honey
- ¾ cup + 3 tablespoons whole almonds, skins on
- 10 eggs, yolks separated from whites
- ¼ tsp salt
- ¼ tsp cream of tartar

For the topping:

- 1 cup double cream
- 1 tbsp. Manuka honey, plus more for drizzling
- A pinch of salt

Directions:

- Preheat the oven to 335 degrees Fahrenheit.
- Grease and line the base of a 9 to 10-inch round tin with parchment paper.
- Cut the butter into small pieces and break up the dark chocolate. Put these in a heatproof bowl, then set this over a pan of simmering water to melt, ensuring that the water does not touch the base of the bowl. Once the butter and chocolate have melted, remove the bowl from the heat and set aside to cool slightly.
- Stir in the Manuka honey. Then, place the almonds in a food processor and blend to a powder. Be careful not to blend them too far because the almonds will release oil if you over process.
- Add the almonds to the chocolate mixture.

- Add the egg yolks to the chocolate mixture one after the other, mixing well after each addition.
- Put the whites in the bowl of a stand mixer with the salt and cream of tartar. Whisk mixture to soft peaks.
- Fold the whites and the chocolate mixture together, and then spoon into the prepared cake tin.
- Bake the cake for 30-35 minutes. The cake should have a slight wobble at its center. Do not over bake it as the gooey richness would be lost.
- Mix the double cream with 1 tbsp. of Manuka honey and the pinch of salt, and then whisk to soft peaks.
- Serve the cake topped with the cream topping and an extra drizzle of Manuka honey. Enjoy!

28. Manuka Honey Catnip Bites

BONUS RECIPENOT for Human Consumption

Ingredients:

- 1 1/2 cups whole wheat flour
- 1 1/2 teaspoons organic catnip
- 1/3 cup dry milk
- 1/2 cup milk
- 2 tablespoons melted butter
- 1 tablespoon Manuka honey
- 1 large egg

Directions:

1. Preheat the oven to 350 degrees Fahrenheit.
2. Combine the dry ingredients in a mixing bowl.
3. Add the wet ingredients and mix with the dry ingredients to form a dough.
4. Roll out the dough and add more flour if needed, and then cut the dough into squares or small shapes.
5. Bake the dough shapes for approximately 20 minutes, or until the treats begin to brown.
6. Let the cat treats cool completely.
7. Store in an airtight container or freeze and thaw as need be. You will have a happy Kitty!

29. Manuka Honey-Mustard Chicken and Potato Casserole

Ingredients:

- 1 pound of potatoes, with skins, sliced lengthwise
- canola oil
- 3 boneless, skinless chicken breasts, cut into thick strips
- 2 medium onions, finely diced
- 5 small sprigs fresh rosemary

<u>Honey Mustard Sauce:</u>

- 2 tablespoons Dijon mustard
- 2 tablespoons grainy mustard
- 1/2 lemon, juiced
- 1 tablespoon canola oil
- 2 tablespoons Manuka honey
- 1/2 cup cream
- 2 cloves garlic, minced
- Olive oil
- Sea salt
- Freshly ground black pepper

Directions:

1. Juice one half of a lemon.
2. Crush the 2 cloves of garlic.

Directions for Manuka Honey-Mustard Chicken and Potato Casserole:

1. Preheat the oven to approximately 390°F.
2. Place a large skillet over medium heat and add 2 tablespoons of canola oil.
3. Stir in the onions and cook for 5 minutes until softened.
4. Remove the skillet from the heat and arrange the potato slices on top in an even layer. Drizzle with olive oil and sprinkle with salt and pepper.
5. Bake in the preheated oven for 20 minutes until softened. Meanwhile, mix the sauce ingredients together in a bowl.
6. Take out the pan from the oven and arrange the strips of raw chicken on top of the potatoes in an even layer. Pour the sauce on top, and make sure everything is coated.
7. Arrange the five sprigs of fresh rosemary around the chicken, cover again with foil, and bake the casserole for 20 minutes. Enjoy!

30. Manuka Honey Ginger Parsnip Bake

Ingredients:

- 1 lb. of parsnip, roughly 4 medium sized
- 2-3 tbsp. butter
- 2 tbsp. Manuka honey
- 3 tbsp. light olive oil
- 1-inch piece of fresh ginger, grated
- Pinch of salt

Directions:

1. Peel the parsnips and cut into match stick shaped pieces.
2. Place parsnip in a single layer in a baking pan.
3. Evenly distribute the Manuka honey, the butter, the oil, the ginger, and the salt over the cut parsnip.
4. Bake on 375°F covered for 40 minutes. Then, uncover, increase temperature to 400 degrees F, and bake for another 10-20 minutes. Serve and Enjoy!

31. Manuka Honey Glazed Pineapple Ham

Ingredients:

- 1 10 pound fully cooked, bone-in ham
- 1 ¼ cups packed dark brown sugar
- 1/3 cup pineapple juice
- 1/3 cup Manuka honey
- 1/3 large orange, juiced and zested
- 2 tablespoons Dijon mustard
- ¼ teaspoon ground cloves

Directions:

Remove the ham from the refrigerator and bring to room temperature, about 30 minutes.

1. Preheat oven to 325 degrees F. Trim off any skin from the ham. Use a sharp paring knife to score through the fat in a diagonal crosshatch pattern without cutting through to the meat.
2. Place ham, flat side down, in a roasting pan. Pour 1/4 inch of water into the bottom of the pan.
3. Transfer ham in the pan to the oven and roast until a thermometer inserted into the thickest part of the ham registers 130 degrees F, which takes about 2 hours and 30 minutes (about 15 minutes per pound).
4. In the meantime, in a small saucepan, combine the brown sugar, pineapple juice, Manuka honey, orange juice, orange zest, Dijon mustard, and ground cloves. Bring to a boil, reduce heat, and simmer for 5 to 10 minutes. Set aside.
5. Bake the ham in the preheated oven uncovered for roughly 2 hours. Remove the ham from oven and brush with glaze. Bake for an additional 30 to 45 minutes, brushing ham with the glaze every 10 minutes. Enjoy!

32. Caramelized Brussel Sprouts with Apples and Pecans

Ingredients:

- 2 tablespoons olive oil, plus additional to finish
- 2 tablespoons butter
- 1 pound of Brussels sprouts, outer leaves removed, quartered
- 1 honey crisp apple, cored, halved, diced
- 3 tablespoons sherry vinegar
- 1 cup pecans, halved, toasted, chopped
- 2-3 tablespoons Manuka honey
- 1/2 cup parsley leaves
- Salt and freshly ground black pepper

Directions:

1. Heat a large cast iron skillet with olive oil and butter over medium-high heat. Add Brussels sprouts, season with salt and pepper, and cook until the sprouts just begin to caramelize, about 4-5 minutes.
2. Add apples and toss to combine, cook until the apples and Brussels sprouts are caramelized and almost tender but still have some firmness, which will take about another 3-4 minutes.
3. Remove from the heat, add the sherry vinegar, pecans, Manuka honey, and parsley. Quickly toss to combine, season with salt and pepper, and remove to a platter. Drizzle with olive oil to finish if you wish. Enjoy!

33. Manuka Honey Fig Dip with Fresh Garlic Pitas

Ingredients:

- 8 oz. cream cheese, softened
- 4 oz. mascarpone cheese, softened
- 8 oz. gorgonzola cheese, crumbled
- 1 cup dried figs, chopped
- 3 tablespoons Manuka honey, plus more for drizzling

For Pitas:

- 6 tablespoons unsalted butter
- 2 garlic cloves, minced
- 6 pita breads
- freshly grated nutmeg
- flaked salt for sprinkling

Directions:

1. Preheat the oven to 375 degrees F.
2. In a bowl, mix together the cream cheese, mascarpone, and gorgonzola with a spatula until creamy and combined.
3. Fold in the figs and Manuka honey, stirring until evenly distributed and combined.
4. Spoon the dip into an oven-safe bowl. Bake for 15 to 20 minutes or until warm and golden on top and bubbly. Top the dip with figs and a decent sized drizzle of Manuka honey as well.
5. While the dip is baking, heat the butter in a small saucepan over medium-low heat and add garlic. Cook just until the butter is bubbling and then remove from the heat.

6. Brush the pitas liberally with the garlic butter. Grate some fresh nutmeg over top, and then sprinkle with flaked sea salt.
7. Slice each pita into 4 or 6 triangles, depending on their size. Place on a baking sheet and stick in the oven for 5 to 6 minutes until just warmed through and fluffy.
8. Serve the fig dip immediately with the warm pitas. Enjoy!

34. Manuka Honey Spiced Carrot Cake

Ingredients:

- 1 ¾ cups all-purpose flour
- 2 teaspoons baking powder
- 1 teaspoon baking soda
- 2 teaspoons ground cinnamon
- 1 teaspoon ground nutmeg
- ½ teaspoon ground cloves
- ½ teaspoon salt
- 1/3 cup plus ¼ cup Manuka honey
- ¾ cup vegetable oil
- 3 large eggs
- 1 tablespoon vanilla extract
- 2 and 2/3 cups shredded carrots

Honey Cream Cheese Frosting (makes about 3 cups)

- 12 ounces cream cheese, softened
- 8 tablespoons unsalted butter, cut into 8 pieces, softened
- 2 teaspoons vanilla extract
- 1/8 teaspoon salt
- 6 tablespoons Manuka honey

Directions for Manuka Honey Carrot Layer Cake:

1. Adjust oven rack to mid position and preheat oven to 350 degrees F. Grease two 9-inch cake pans, line with parchment paper, grease parchment, and flour the pans.
2. Whisk flour, baking powder, baking soda, cinnamon, nutmeg, cloves, and salt together in one bowl.

3. In another bowl, whisk Manuka honey, oil, eggs, and vanilla together until smooth. Stir in shredded carrots. Add flour mixture and fold with a rubber spatula until combined.
4. Divide batter evenly among pans, smoothing the tops. Bake until cakes are set, and their centers are firm to touch, about 15 to 20 minutes.
5. Rotate pans halfway through baking. Let cakes cool 10 minutes, then remove from pans. Discard parchment and allow cakes to cool completely on a rack for one hour.
6. Spread one cup of frosting over first cake layer and add second cake layer, pressing evenly to adhere. Spread one cup frosting over top and remaining frosting over the sides.

Honey Cream Cheese Frosting: Using stand mixer with whisk attachment, whip the cream cheese, butter, vanilla, and salt on medium-high speed until smooth, about 1 to 2 minutes. Reduce mixer speed to medium-low and whip frosting until light and fluffy, about 3 to 5 minutes. Enjoy!

35. Manuka Honey and Thyme Cornbread

Ingredients:

- 1 ½ cups yellow cornmeal
- ½ cup all-purpose flour
- 2 teaspoons baking powder
- 1 teaspoon salt
- ½ teaspoon baking soda
- 2 eggs
- 2 cups sour cream
- 2 tablespoons Manuka honey
- 1 tablespoon fresh thyme leaves
- 1 tablespoon rendered bacon fat or coconut oil

Directions:

1. Preheat the oven to 450 degrees F.
2. In a large bowl, whisk together the dry ingredients (cornmeal, flour, baking powder, and salt).
3. In a separate bowl, beat the eggs, and then whisk in the sour cream.
4. Fold the sour cream and eggs into the dry ingredient mixture until fully blended and cohesive.
5. Stir in the Manuka honey and thyme.
6. Melt the bacon fat (or coconut oil) in the skillet and coat the bottom. Pour any excess into the batter and stir.
7. Pour batter into a 10-inch skillet and bake for 15 to 20 minutes or until browned at the top and a toothpick inserted in the center comes out clean.
8. Wait to cool or serve hot and fresh as a side dish or a snack. Enjoy!

36. Manuka Honey Raspberry Bundt Cake

Ingredients:

For the Cake:

- 1 cup (2 sticks) unsalted butter, softened
- 2 cups Manuka honey
- 2 teaspoons vanilla
- zest from one lemon
- 6 large eggs
- 2 cups whole wheat flour
- 2 cups all-purpose flour
- 1/2 teaspoon baking soda
- 1/2 teaspoon kosher salt
- 1 cup plain yogurt, NOT GREEK YOGURT
- 2 cups fresh raspberries

For the Glaze:

- 2 tablespoons Manuka honey
- 2 tablespoons milk
- 1 cup confectioners' sugar

Directions:

1. Preheat the oven to 350 degrees F. Spray a 10-inch tube pan or a 12-cup Bundt pan with cooking spray.
2. Beat the butter and Manuka honey together in the bowl of a stand mixer at medium/low until the mixture is smooth and a pale color that is almost white, which will take about 3 minutes.

3. Beat in the vanilla and lemon zest. Add the eggs, one at a time, beating well after each addition. The mixture may look curdled, this is OK.

4. Beat in the flours, baking soda, and salt one cup at a time, alternating with the yogurt, until the batter is smooth and well blended. Gently fold in 1-1/2 cups of the raspberries using a spatula or a spoon.

5. Place several of the remaining berries in the bottom of the prepared pan and spoon the batter over them. Spread the batter out evenly to fill the pan, then press the remaining raspberries into the top of the batter.

6. Bake for 45–50 minutes or until the cake pulls away from the sides of the pan and a tester inserted in the center comes out clean. Let cool in the pan on a rack for 10 minutes, and then invert onto a serving platter.

For the glaze: Beat the milk and Manuka honey together in a medium-sized bowl, and then add the confectioners' sugar until you have a spoon able glaze. Drizzle over the cake, creating an even layer on top and let it drip down the sides of the cake some for decoration. Enjoy!

37. Vanilla and Manuka Honey Homemade Ice Cream

Ingredients:

- 6 large egg yolks
- ½ cup granulated sugar
- ⅓ cup Manuka honey
- 2 teaspoons vanilla extract
- ¼ teaspoon fine sea salt
- 3 cups heavy cream
- 3 ounces of cream cheese, cubed, at room temperature
- ⅓ cup whole milk

Directions:

In a large bowl, whisk together yolks, sugar, Manuka honey, vanilla, and salt until smoothly blended.

1. In a medium saucepan over medium heat, bring heavy cream to a simmer.
2. Whisking the yolks constantly, slowly pour half of the hot cream into the egg mixture.
3. Scrape custard back into saucepan and cook over medium-low heat, stirring constantly, until the custard is thick enough to coat the back of a spoon (about 180 degrees on an instant-read thermometer). Do not let mixture come to a simmer, as it could curdle.
4. Strain into a heatproof bowl and whisk in cream cheese until completely melted.
5. Set the bowl in a larger bowl filled with ice water.

6. Using a hand mixer or an immersion blender, whip custard until thick and cold for about 5 minutes. Then, spoon mixture into 3 or 4 ice cube trays, and freeze for at least 3 hours or overnight.
7. Using an offset spatula or a butter knife, pop out ice cream cubes.
8. Transfer to a food processor or a blender. Pulse cubes with whole milk until the ice cream is smooth and has the consistency of soft serve. Serve immediately or return to container and freeze. Enjoy!

39334612R00036

Printed in Poland
by Amazon Fulfillment
Poland Sp. z o.o., Wrocław